Bellydance Bliss

A Woman's Unique Guide to Self-Fulfillment

Lorran Wild

Balboa Press books may be ordered through booksellers or by contacting:

Balboa Press
A Division of Hay House
1663 Liberty Drive
Bloomington, IN 47403
www.balboapress.com
1 (877) 407-4847

ISBN: 978-1-4525-1999-9 (sc)
ISBN: 978-1-4525-2000-1 (e)

Library of Congress Control Number: 2014914535

Printed in the United States of America.

Balboa Press rev. date: 12/02/2014

BALBOA.
PRESS
A DIVISION OF HAY HOUSE

Bellydance Bliss

A Woman's Unique Guide to Self-Fulfillment

Contents

APPENDIX

Acknowledgements

Dance is a gift:

A teacher, a medicine, a lover, a child, a prayer.

Dance is a magic carpet to ride to other worlds, other realities
and other possibilities.

Dance is a path:

A gateway to transformation.

My whole life's a dance swirling through time and place.

I entreat you to dance

Discover the wisdom of your body

Foster your love for the feminine in women

Lorran (.)

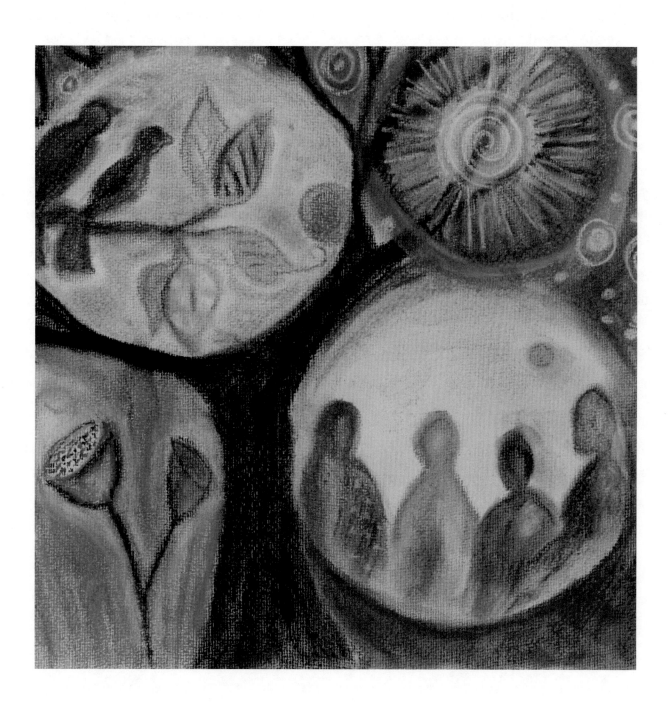

Preface

When I approached the door to my first bellydance class, I had fear and doubt. I wondered who else would be there and if we would get along. I wondered why I was interested in something I had never seen or done before. As I got closer, I planned my exit in case I was asked to go topless. But I also felt brave and hopeful. I was longing for fun and community. I was searching for a way to love myself and my womanhood.

I was searching for an experience of fulfilment.

As I walked down the hallway, it was the music that drew me in. Breathy flute and captivating rhythms beckoned to me. That first class was unforgettable. The women were all shapes and sizes, all ages and stages of life; not a typical dance class. My heart danced with grace and joy!

The movements were hard to do, but they gave me pleasure from beginning. I'm sure I did sweat, but that wasn't important. I glowed! My fondest memory is the feeling of belonging and the sound of our laughter. I became entranced. Before I went to bed each night, I danced. In fact, I could not sleep soundly without it.

The dance became my medicine, my art, my teacher, my lover and my creation.

For over 20 years, I studied, taught and performed in 'The Art of Middle Eastern Dance'. However, what I discovered was that this dance was more global and universal than cultural. I learned that Bellydance is for every woman, not just the pretty woman or the fit woman or the brown woman or the 'whatever' woman.

Using This Book

This book is not a fitness manual (even though you might get in great shape). You may choose to add a training routine and suitable nutrition into your day for building strength and stamina. These exercises are intended to nurture your creativity. Connecting your body, feelings and thoughts into a dance is the ultimate purpose of this practice.

The dance poems are meant for your inspiration, not intended as dance instruction. Chapters 1-9 are designed to help you develop a home practice of dancing. In Chapter 10, there are some suggestions for creating social dance gatherings. The Appendix has musical suggestions for each chapter.

Please go at your own pace. Bellydance Bliss takes time and patient practice. Each day you dance is like a day in the garden. You must actively await the germination and ripening of the seeds you plant, making sure they have the right conditions for blossom and fruit. One day, you will harvest wisdom from your care and attention...just like the generations of women before you.

It is worth reading through the entire chapter before you put on the music and try it out. You may be tempted to get someone to read it to you while you dance, or record yourself. However, these are not meditations. They are inspirations. Read through them and then dance, trusting that you will remember what you need for the moment. Read over them again and again. Dance each section again and again. One day, you will come to your practice with a sense of trust that your body will tell you what to do. The dance is ultimately your true guide.

...Let Intuition Guide You...

Introduction

O keep squeezing drops of the Sun
From your prayers and work and music
And from your companions' beautiful laughter
And from the most insignificant movements
Of your own holy body.
Now, sweet one, be wise.
Cast all your votes for Dancing!

~Hafiz

Ancient Origins

Bellydance is rooted in the soil of women's collective experience. Within that 'garden of life' blossomed sacred movements: dances of worship, birth and love. In the daily activities of work, there was a dance. In the mystery of their soul was a dance. The circular strength of stirring the pot grew into dance movements. The subtle gestures of love-making became sacred in their dance. Every life-honouring event, from babies born and youth coming of age, to the passing of loved ones; bellydance was a core part of every celebration.

However, through many centuries of endeavor,
the bouquet of bellydance lost some of its roots
and changed its purpose, from a spiritual practice
into an entertainment.

Eternal Wisdom Dances in You

Today, women are drawn to learn the ancient techniques of bellydance to socialize with each other; move their body in flowing and gentle ways and connect to something eternal about themselves. Entering a class often has the experience of being familiar, yet exotic. The hypnotic qualities of the movements soothe and calm a restless body and soul. Yet, as multitudes of women attend bellydance class and learn to enjoy the movements of their bodies, they often sense that something essential is missing within the choreography.

This book offers the essence of a woman's dance practice that is both ancient and eternal. The original women's dance was not about performance or culture. It was a path to learning about being feminine in the most sacred way. With a regular practice and study of bellydance, every woman connects to an ancient lineage. There is an ancient feminine voice that speaks through us when we bellydance. Every woman has an inner wisdom that is derived by moving intuitively.

If we seek the real source of the dance,
if we go to nature,
we find that the dance of the future
is the dance of the past, the dance of eternity,
and has been and will always be the same."

~Isadora Duncan

Cultural Perceptions

Contrary to limiting perceptions which might suggest a specific country of origin, bellydance does not belong to a certain culture (unless you are performing with the intention of representation). Bellydance is a universal and global dance for the female body. Anywhere you go on earth, the dance of life is cradled within the belly of women. Bellydance is their dance.

Cultures of the world including Hawaii, Polynesia, India, Spain, Latin America, Africa and First Nations; all share movements for women which radiate from the lower belly and involve free movement of the hips.

Bellydance offers a woman access to body awareness and wisdom, regardless of her cultural origins. Through the dance, we can share in each other's traditions and transcend any inherited limitations.

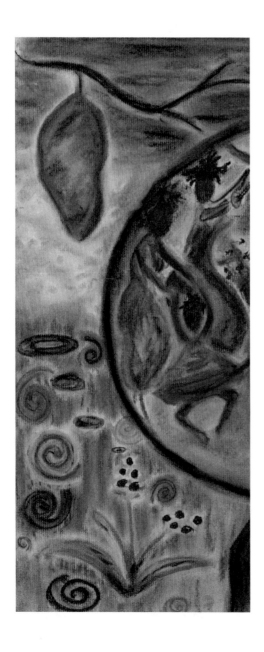

So dance, little sister, Dance...
for as long as you Dance,
this ancient women's wisdom
will live and grow,
unfurling its red thread to all
the daughters
of earth and heaven.

Your Body is a Masterpiece

By doing the exercises in this book in the privacy of your chamber, you will cultivate a moving practice that will teach you, nourish you, pleasure you and heal you. This kind of practice is Dance with a capital 'D'. Dance becomes a sanctuary where you unite with your true essence, unfettered by culture or circumstance; divinely spiritual and blissfully earthly. You do not get lost in the Dance. Like entering a labyrinth, you take yourself back to your centre; and feel a sense of 'home' as you go back out into the world.

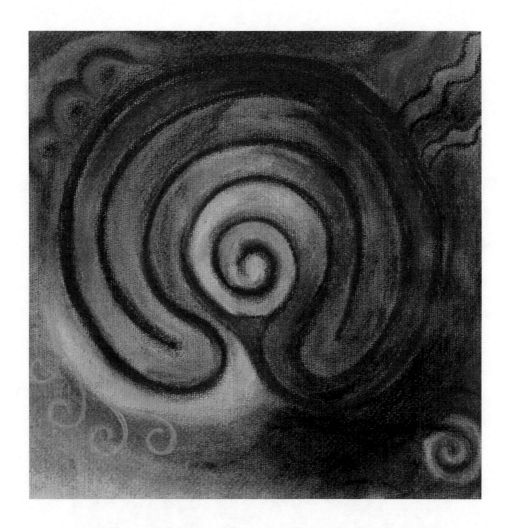

"The moment in between what you once were,
and who you are now becoming,
is where the dance of life really takes place."

~Barbara de Angelis

Creating Space

Having a home 'studio' space is essential to making dance a part of your daily lifestyle. Claim a space somewhere in your home: basement, bedroom, living room. It doesn't need to be a full room, but take as much space as you can and own it. A beautiful and spacious area of your home dedicated to your movement practice is invaluable. It becomes a sanctuary. You can go there to let your emotions dance, your dreams dance, your prayers dance, and your body dance. Create your space for safety, beauty, freedom, and warmth. Use your favorite fabrics, colors and candles.

If the *body* is the temple of *the spirit,* surely its most exalted use is *Dance*

~DeAnn

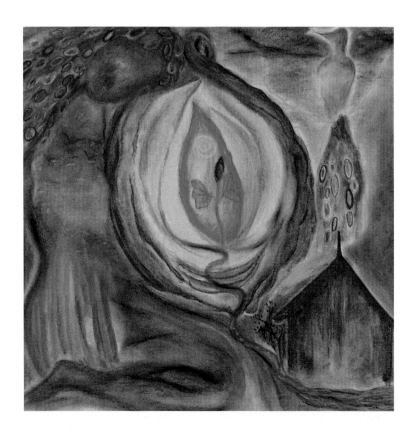

Practice versus Training

The guidance here seeks to inspire you to move beyond the class experience and deepen your relationship to your own glorious body through the wisdom of bellydance. In conventional exercise programs, you are training the body for strength and endurance. The goal of a training regime is to exhaust muscles and push the limits of the body. Panting and sweating are favorable indicators of success during a workout.

Your Dance is Your Pleasure

Bellydance is not a sport or aerobic 'workout'. Bellydance is a practice. The purpose is to make the body radiate with bliss. The dancer may perspire, but that is not the goal. Success is measured in release of tension, deepened breathing, soothed muscles and organs, limbered joints and smiles.

Pleasure is WILD and *sweet*.
She likes purple flowers.
She loves the sun and the wind and the night sky.
She carries a silver bowl full of liquid moonlight.
She has a cat named Midnight with stars on his paws.
Many people mistrust Pleasure, and even more misunderstand her.
For a long time I could barely stand to be in ...the same room with her..."

— J. Ruth Gendler, ***The Book of Qualities***

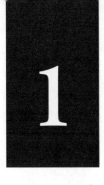

Feminine Wisdom:
Roots of Women's Power

In an effort to establish equality between men and women, we have been jeopardizing a very important aspect of our humanity. Women now contribute to new spheres of power, such as positions of leadership and decision-making, but in order to do this, we often diminish much of our femininity, dismissing it as 'stupid', 'silly' and 'trivial'- a grave mistake. True equality is not about sameness. It is about balance. There is a difference between the masculine and the feminine, and both are necessary for the well-being of humanity. If we lose femininity in the wake of feminism, we are, in effect, killing an essential aspect of our humanity. The terrible consequences range from neglected children to reproductive disorders.

The World of Humanity has 2 wings
One is Feminine, the other Masculine
Only when both wings are strong
Will the bird be capable of flight

~Baha'u'llah

Femininity is not a weakness. As we will see with the archetypes, the feminine power is a motivational leader. Where the strength of the masculine lies in protecting, providing and producing, the strength of the feminine is in revealing, receiving and reflecting. Through balance, a reciprocal harmony is established between the polarities, and each is enhanced.

It's about equal value, not sameness

We all have a full spectrum of masculine and feminine attributes. However, the DNA of male-ness or female-ness creates very real distinctions in a man and a woman. Besides the obvious physical characteristics, there are other, more subtle instincts that develop. A woman more strongly develops the hormones and physiology for the diffuse awareness needed for gathering herbaceous plants, staying alert to predators, and minding children. This means she also has an awareness of subtle emotions, side conversations and things that are 'out of place'. A man generally develops the hormones and physiology for the focused thinking necessary to stalk and attack. This means his instincts can focus on a question, a television show or a task without diverting his attention on other things (even if those other things are actually more important to him).

This is not to say that women can't hunt, or that men can't take care of children. Each individual is a unique blueprint of DNA and has a spectrum of natural propensities.

Take pudding and ice cream as a metaphor. Both are made from cream, eggs and sugar, but once you cool them to setting, they cannot be reversed or changed into becoming the other. Both are delicious, but when you want ice cream, pudding will not do. Likewise, there are many different recipes and flavours to create within each one. They are both 'dessert', but there are many differences. A woman will never be a man. A man will never be a woman. They are both human. One is like pudding. One is like ice cream. Women are valuable for their way of being. Men are valuable for their way of being. Negating or oppressing one does not increase the value of the other.

"The intuitive mind is a sacred gift
and the rational mind is a faithful servant.
We have created a society that honours the servant
and has forgotten the gift."

~Albert Einstein

Connect to your Femininity

As we learn to consciously embrace and balance the elemental forces and tensions that constitute our full-spectrum humanity, we actually generate new capacities and possibilities. Becoming more masculine is not strengthening to women or the world we love. It makes us tired and lonely. In fact, the strain on our adrenals from the demands for testosterone in our production-driven world is causing tremendous fatigue and chronic disease. It would be wiser to educate and remind each other about the contributions made by the feminine so that we can establish a true equality - one based in the strengths of each, not in sameness. There is courage in being vulnerable. There is strength in softness.

Hence, as we transition from a world that requests a woman to produce, protect and provide, into a world that values more feminine qualities, women need to claim time to rebalance themselves and reconnect with their authentic femininity in some way.

"Within every woman, there is a *Wild* and Natural creature, a *powerful force*, filled with good instincts, *passionate creativity*, and *ageless knowing*. Her name is *Wild Woman*, but she is an endangered species."

~Clarissa Pinkola Estes-(Women Who Run With The Wolves).

It takes courage to be vulnerable: be Brave

To cultivate femininity, you need to connect with the qualities of RECEPTIVITY. Being receptive means honouring yourself, your observations, your feelings and intuition, your wants and needs, your cycles and changes. Being feminine is strong, yet voluntarily vulnerable. It takes courage to reveal yourself; ask for what makes you glorious.

This is not easy. In an effort to adapt to our times, and succeed in life, many women have given up on being true to themselves. We may feel as though we need to provide more, or prove something. Often, the connection to our femininity is so diminished that we cannot even identify with what (exactly) we want to do, be, feel and have.

> *"I want to think again*
> *of dangerous and noble things.*
> *I want to be light and frolicsome.*
> *I want to be the improbable and beautiful*
> *and afraid of nothing as though I had wings."*
>
> *~Mary Oliver*

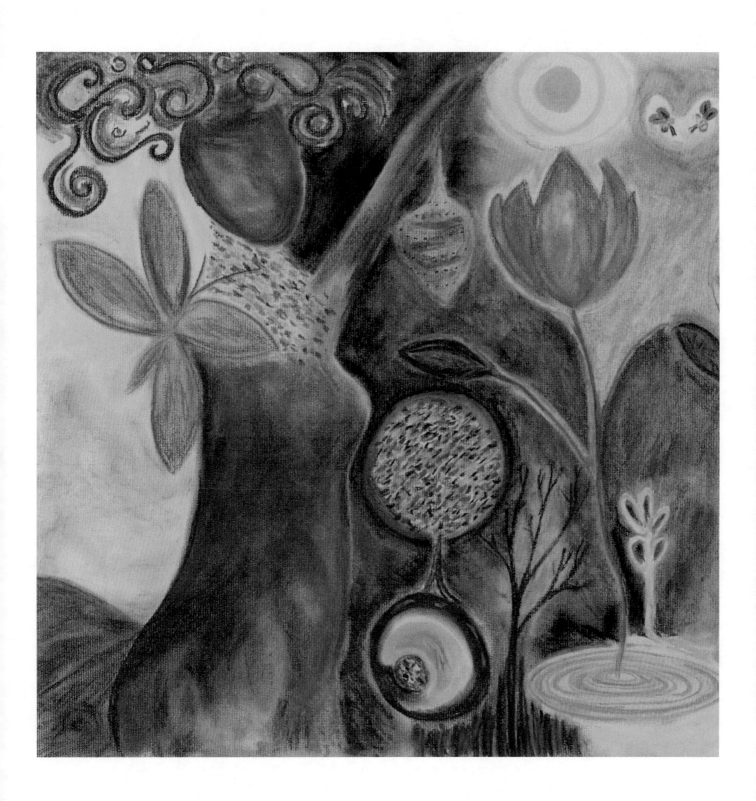

Dance of Femininity

This is a dance that awakens sensual warmth in the body. Very simply, you will put on some melodic, sensual music...

Stand with your eyes closed
focus your attention between the fleshiest parts of your inner thighs
(not the vagina, but just below it)
Once you have a sensation of warmth,
begin to move as you maintain ITA (inner thigh awareness)

Your knees and ankles soften
your head lilts upon your neck,
your hips rock and sway,
your arms undulate and float

Now bring your attention to your heart
The temple of your feelings
Move from the sensations that arise here
Allow the warmth of your thighs to rise up
And the sensation of the heart to draw downwards
To meet in your belly
Breathing softness; Revealing beauty; Receiving healing
Blossoming into Creativity and Love

N.B. You can connect with ITA anytime and anywhere. It's a good start to arousing your femininity, but be careful about dancing with it in public, because you may get more attention than you want to handle!

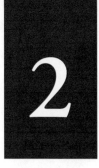

Invoke the Senses:
Gateways of Self-Fulfilment

To understand your body; to hear its subtle messages of pleasure and pain; to reclaim the intuitive knowing of what you need to heal and be well; you need to be intimate with your anatomy.

It is assumed you are familiar with the location of major organs involved in digestion and circulation such as stomach, liver, spleen, heart, lung, intestine, etc. If you are not, a quick visit to the library or the internet will provide you with this information. Whenever you have internal pain, it is worthwhile information to have.

For the purposes of dancing, this chapter will describe the sensory organs. The senses of seeing, hearing, touch, taste and smell are the keys to a woman's sensuality. Once you know how to nourish your senses, you are on the path of fulfilment. The senses are the conduit between worlds. They are the receivers of impressions in the realm of spirit and earth.

In moving the body through bellydance, the senses come alive. The blood flows warmly to the skin. In dance, you radiate with life and happiness. There is no elixir more captivating than a happy and sensuous woman!

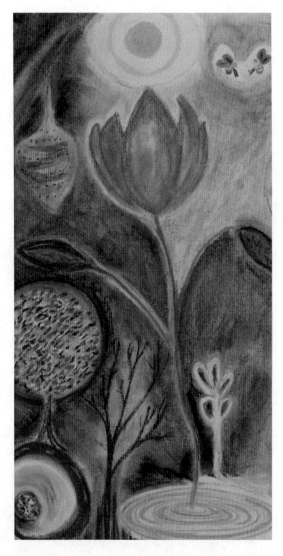

Studies show that people who are especially sensual have a tendency to be more 'present'. They are not living in the past, projecting the future; they are in a state of 'oneness'. There is opportunity in sensuality to slow down and pay full attention to the feeling at hand; an opportunity to bask in the actual moment of sensuality rather than rush through life.

Immerse yourself in the pleasures of the senses

Sensuality is not sexuality. It is the special ingredient of fulfilment in all life. It improves the sexual experience, but not because they are the same thing. Sensuality has to do with enjoying the pleasure of your senses: sight, smell, sound, taste and touch. It's about being awakened and stimulated by things that activate these various senses.

To have sensuality is to be aware of, appreciate and take delight in our senses. It is to live a life felt through our senses. When we shift focus from thinking, into that which is felt, seen, smelled, touched, heard and tasted, it has a significant and positive bearing on how we experience life.

Giving special care and attention to the organs of sensation is a worthwhile activity any time of day. It is good preparation for your dancing practice. It is also a wonderful way to close your session and transition into the next part of your day. Schedule time to nourish and pamper at least one of your senses every day.

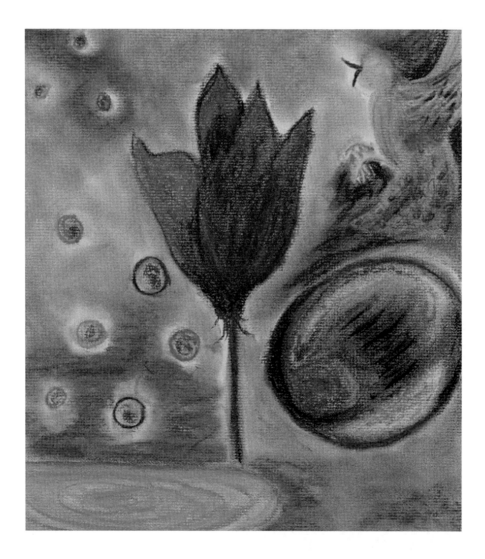

Seeing

The eyes are known as the 'mirror of the soul' and the 'ocean of spirit'. Through our gaze we communicate thoughts and feelings. Even someone who is avoiding our glance is revealing something.

Try this:

Looking into a mirror
Observe directly your eyes
See the depth, the liveliness, the questions
Now try to stir up different emotions or moods
Joy
Anger
Sorrow
Kindness
Resistance
Love
See how your eyes are transformed...

Vision is not limited to what the eyes perceive. The dancer who sees with her eyes closed is accessing other senses of perception such as touch and hearing, but she is also gazing inward. This is a good way of creating space for insight.

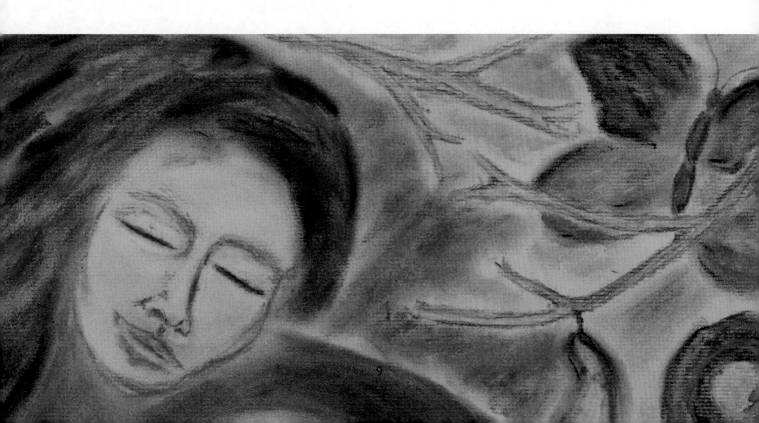

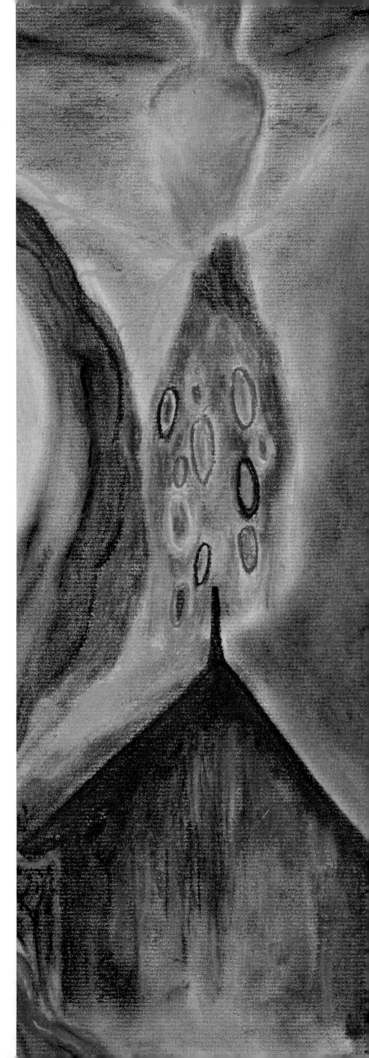

Dance of Sight

Whenever you are dancing, take some time to gaze in different directions and distances. Look directly in various places, stare into the distance. Open them wide or half-close them. Play with different moods: shy, demanding, worried, and confident. Notice how it changes your dance experience.

Begin dancing with your eyes closed

Moving in space as much as you dare

At some point, open your eyes and gaze at what is before you

Roll your eyes around every direction (without moving your head)

Stretch their muscles

Then close your eyes again

In your mind, recreate what you saw

Close your eyes again

Move to another location – 'blinded'

Guided by your body's sensual way of 'seeing' – inner sight

Open your eyes and gaze about you

With your eyes, send a message to what you see

Alternate your looking and closing eyes until you are satisfied

Hearing

If the eyes are the 'mirror of the soul', then the ears are the 'gateway to the soul'. The ears are designed like a shell so that sounds spiral into the body. Unpleasant sounds affect our mood in negative ways. Favorable sounds can uplift our spirits and bring us peaceful moods.

So important is our hearing! The very act of listening takes a special activity in the brain. Unlike the eyes which form pictures directly through the cornea, sounds must be taken and transposed from waves and oscillations, into a 'sound picture'. Hearing is the first sense to develop; the ears emerge *in utero* on the seventh or eighth day. Four and a half months later, the internal ear has reached its final size, giving a fetus considerable auditory experience! At the moment of death, when all our senses fade away, when we no longer feel, taste or smell, our hearing lingers the longest.

Furthermore, our hearing sense is also critical for balance. The nerve network linking the ear to the spine is denser than the one linking the eye. In order to stand or walk upright, the ear must receive information from balance receptors located throughout the body, down to the soles of the feet. When you fall, a contraction is provoked by the internal ear, which prevents the back of the head from hitting the ground and sets the point of impact on the spine, near the center of gravity. Observe yourself; when you want to hearken to a sound, your body straightens up.

Listening Dance

Choose a song that has pauses of silence in it.
Melody plays
Dance with it
Take the music into the body and make it visible
In the pause of silence
Be still and focus within
The dance of sensations you are feeling
Skin
Organs
Thoughts
Moods
When the melody returns
Stay in stillness and continue to hearken to what dances within
When the silence comes again
Dance a silent dance in praise of what has moved in you

Try this:

Put on some music and rub your ears with your hands
Stand in a basic position
Start circling your hips, and put your hands on your belly
Let the music flow into your ears and guide it along a spiral, all the way down to your belly

Connect your ears to your belly,
as it is gently massaged by your circling hips
Fill your pelvis with music;
Let it flow and submerge you
Feel the music as it fills up your body

How do your ears feel? Your belly? Is it changing into a resounding surface for all sounds, all rhythms, relaying them to your whole body?

Can you perceive how it is possible to see with your ears and listen
with your eyes?

And what then is silence?
Could it be the impulse that transforms utterance into form?

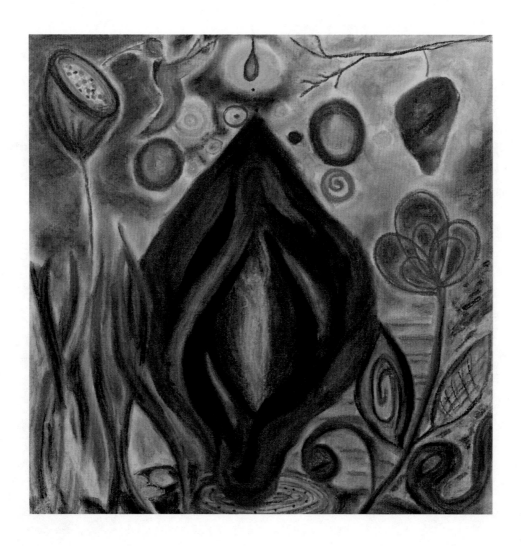

This is meditation; the pause between breaths
the melodic wisdom of the universe.
Each sound returns to silence.
Silence is the origin;
the place where the soul can dance.

Smell

As human beings, we are emotionally impacted by scent. In fact, our sense of smell is considered the only sense that evokes a purely emotional response. Research indicates that smells are not filtered through the part of the brain that ruminates or analyzes, but rather though the part that responds and operates without conscious thought. It is reported that our responses to smell take place within ten seconds after exposure — with no thought process involved. We react, and then think.

Not only do certain smells affect how we feel emotionally, but they can also affect our energy level. Overly strong perfumes can invoke irritation and revolt. The aroma of delicious food can entice pleasurable feelings of well-being.

Aromatherapy is a therapy which uses essential oils as remedies. (pure and natural essential oils only...synthetic scents are pollutants). They are used in massaging the skin, but their potency enters through the nose. Here are some common oils and their uses:

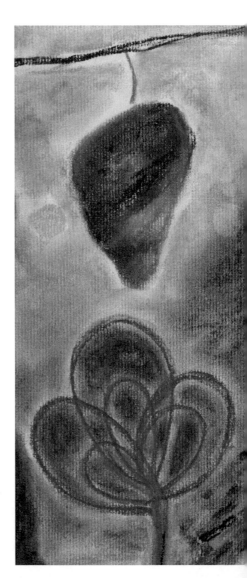

For calm: chamomile or lavender

To be more alert: rosemary, peppermint, eucalyptus or lemongrass

For amorous encounters: ylang-ylang, sandalwood, rose and jasmine are for a sensual bedroom; vanilla, neroli and lavender awakens your sensuality.

Try this:

Take yourself and a daughter, sister or friend
Go on a 'sensual date'
find a shopping location where there will be lots of different smells; some kind of candle vendor,
food market
or body care shop are excellent choices.
Do a bit of sense exploration;
sample lotions and potions,
do some taste tests
gaze at the beauty
Discover what is pleasing to your senses.
When you are done walking around, find a cafe and have a treat!

Dance of Scent

Light a scented candle,
oil diffuser
or a stick of incense in a corner of the room
(aim for pure and natural essential oils for your health)
While gentle music plays, begin your dance in an opposite corner
Using beckoning gestures
Swaying
Swirling
Dance as the fragrance is wafting throughout the room
Use your movement to bring it into your body
through your sense of smell
Pay attention to when you can first smell it
As the smell intensifies, allow your dance to intensify
As the smell dissipates, allow your dance to ease

Touch Dance

With a length of silk fabric, in a safe and comfortable place where you are completely alone (bedroom or bathroom perhaps), remove all of your clothes:

Begin humming sounds to yourself and wrap yourself into the silk
Move and sway with your humming
Paying attention to the sensations on your skin
Use the silk as if you were anointing yourself with oil
Feel your hair; your face; your neck
Allow the silk to caress your hands, trace down your arms and torso; your legs and feet
Dance the silk into the air
Can you feel the breath of it on your skin?

Try this:

When you feel tired, when your head gets heavy and your connection to your body feels weak, sit down and give your feet a massage. Better yet, soak your feet in a warm footbath and rub them with oil while you listen to soothing music. You'll see how, after such a massage, your feet will carry you more sensitively.

Let your naked feet dance with you
Your toes wiggle and spread
Roll through the entire arch; from heel to ball
Walk by touching the heel first
Then walk by touching the toes first
Stamp on the floor
Rub the ground with your whole foot
Trace patterns with your big toe
Play with new ways of traveling
Then lie on your back and let your feet dance and play in the air
Have fun with your soles!

Taste

Nature has endowed animals with the sense of taste to aid their survival. What tastes sour or bitter is usually poisonous and better avoided. Sweet flavors are normally nourishing.

Food is an integral component to the sense of taste, but it is also a metaphor for good living. Consider phrases such as; "It's all a matter of taste", "That encounter left a bitter taste", "Savour the sweetness of life". Such phrases open up the horizons of taste beyond the scope of survival, into a sensual experience.

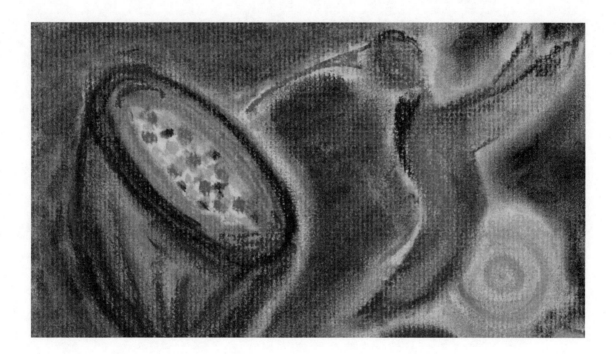

Dance of Taste

Here is where food comes in. Yay! Create a loving tray of delectable treats: luscious fruits, creamy delights, luxurious sweets and savory indulgences.

While the music plays:

Cup your face
Massage your mouth with your fingers
Stroke your hair
Rub your belly
Let the weight shift through your legs and hips
in rocking and swaying patterns
At any moment, choose a morsel of food
Smell it, touch it and gaze at it for a breath or two before you
put it in your mouth
Get in touch with the way it tastes
Roll on the floor as you savour the flavour, the texture
Let it dance inside your mouth
Feel the gratitude for your senses and the nourishment of food
Continue savouring the taste of this dance,
even after the food is all gone.

3

Wisdom of Archetypes

In ancient times, cultural decisions were guided by initiates who created an elaborate oral tradition about gods and goddesses. Their insight was regarded as spiritual authority and followed as a religion. We may no longer be willing to make faithful offerings at the temple of Aphrodite to mend our marriage, or ask Durga to protect us in a battle; but the attributes of ancient goddesses are a mirror of truth; reflecting a core of our deepest qualities. If we distill the feminine archetypes into their simplest manifestations, we have the Temptress, Mother and Queen. A woman can embody these archetypes simultaneously at any stage of life. They are not separate in our identity, but form a dynamic wholeness.

"How could we forget those ancient myths
that stand at the beginning of all races,
the myths about dragons
that at the last moment
are transformed into princesses?
Perhaps all the dragons in our lives are princesses
who are only waiting to see us act, just once,
with beauty and courage."

~ Rainer Maria Rilke

Temptress: The Temptress is largely a physical aspect of womanhood. Here is the part of us that is playful, fun-loving and giggly. The Temptress attracts laughter and skipping. Others are drawn into her playful spirit and joyful ways. She is not a vixen or sex object, although she loves to come out when we are in love.

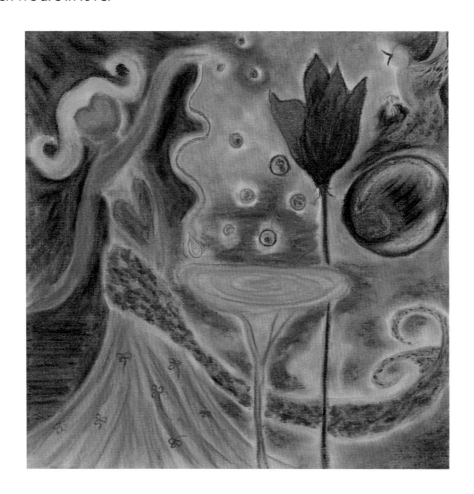

Dance with the Temptress

Find music that entices you to put a bounce or skip
in your step. With a length of silky fabric in your
hands (an appealing color is recommended):
Trace round and curvy shapes in the air,
on the floor,
on your body.
Touch and tease the room and its contents,
as if everything in it was a playmate.
Touch yourself in ways that tickle out the giggles.
Find the pleasure of being yourself,
Free-spirited

Mother: Contrary to 'mothering', which is a distorted and depleted version of a woman who asserts power over those she loves by demanding, manipulating and forcing obedience to her authority; the Mother archetype is a potent source of healing and wellness. When we are in the archetype of the Mother, we love unconditionally and offer nourishment and rest as a solution for ailments of all kinds. The Mother listens without trying to solve problems; giving comfort in hugs and smiles; patiently loving us until we find our way. She expects no reward; has no need for appreciation, praise or approval. The Mother is the archetype for the emotional and nurturing aspect of womanhood.

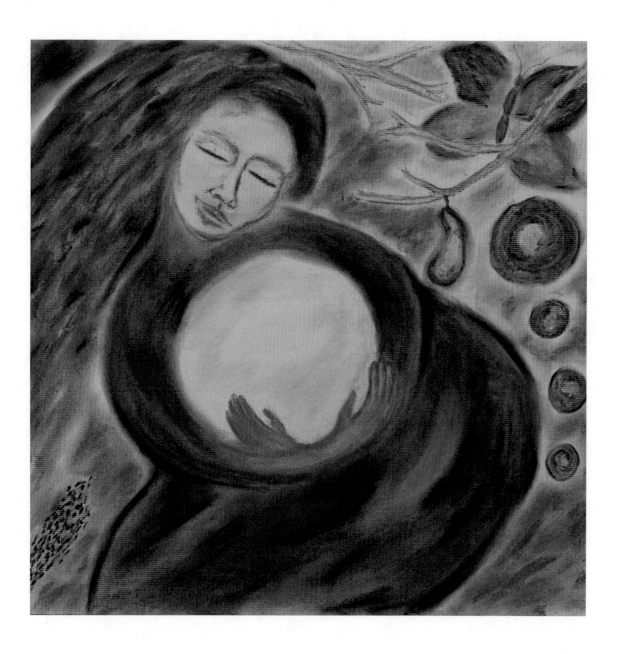

Dance with the Mother

Put on soothing music that has a woman's voice you love to hear. Lullabies are great for this (see appendix). Light a candle (or many if you wish). Make sure there is safety and comfort. This light represents you and the Mother archetype.

Gather other symbols of the Mother such as: tea service, cup of warm milk, a grain/seed treat, fresh fruit, hair brush, shawl, etc. Place them around your space.

Hold and caress yourself in a loving way
Let your hands rub your heart
Allow your worries and cares to nestle in your arms
You are absolutely beautiful, just as you are
Visit each of the stations you have created
Take up the symbol you have placed there and use it
To give and receive love
To nurture and nourish
To cherish and behold
Dance with the lilt of the music
as if you are both divine mother and divine child

You Are...

To close this dance, take up some colours and paper and draw an image of the mother – full, round, generous, loving , beautiful.

Queen: Here is the archetype that inspires nobility and heroism. The Queen prevails in the spiritual aspects of womanhood. It is she who has an extraordinary ability to receive, be generous, gracious and serene. Bringing out the archetype of the Queen takes some finesse and lots of practice because she is not expressed by our instincts and there aren't many role models to show us the way. The Queen has defined boundaries and clear perspective. She can make requests and knowingly ask for her needs, without depending on others. She doesn't need to be rescued. She allows others to help her because she deeply understands that giving and receiving bring out the best in humanity.

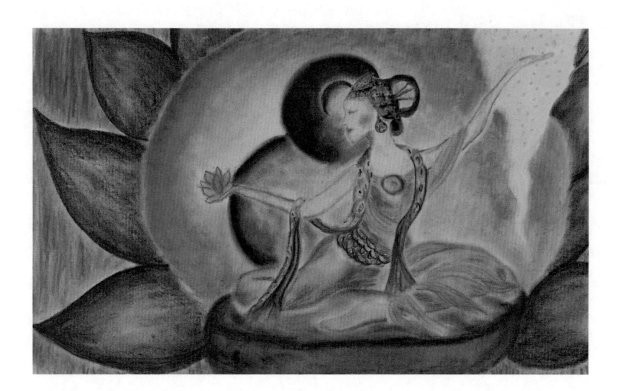

Dance with the Queen

Do you have a crown?
What do you wear to feel noble and full of grace?
How could you connect with your spiritual aspects?

Adorn yourself with a raiment that invokes the Queen in you.

To dance with the spirit of Queen, you will move without any music:

Go into the silence and dance your prayers.
Spread your offerings, your hopes and dreams
through your blood and bones,
into the space that surrounds you.
Feel them carried on your breath to the Infinite Mystery

Notice your hands
Gaze at them while they sculpt the air and search for the messages communicated there

After completing this chapter, take a moment to reflect on yourself:

Which goddess aspect do you find easy to be?
Which aspects have been absent or neglected?

Are you *healed* in Her arms?

Are you saved in Her grace?

Are you *waked* in Her love?

Are you *found* in Her light?

~Janin Canan

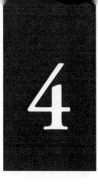

Dance in Beauty

One of the biggest lessons in bellydance is to make a distinction between 'pretty' and 'beautiful'. 'Pretty' is a culmination of genetics and personal fashion. 'Beautiful' is cultivated by eternal qualities such as inner strength, love, passion, courage, generosity and honesty.

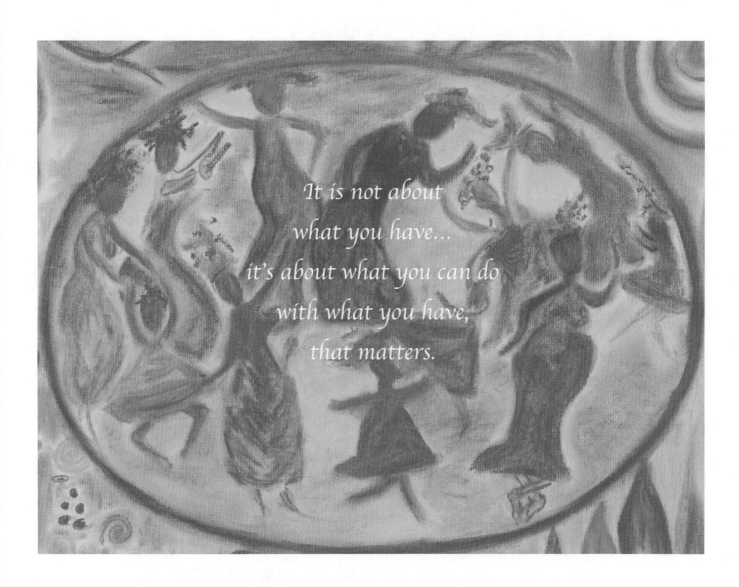

It is not about
what you have...
it's about what you can do
with what you have,
that matters.

Pretty dance does not touch the heart and soul; it mostly causes competition, jealousy and low self-esteem. Dance that reveals our beauty inspires and bestirs the heart and soul. It causes transformation and joy.

To connect with Beauty, a bellydancer learns to isolate every body part. This facilitates the muscular control necessary to make the nuances of music visible through dance. However, there is another benefit to learning isolations. When the attention moves from one body part to the next, there comes an awareness and appreciation for the beauty that is revealed there. For example, if you witness your own hands as they sculpt the space and respond to music, you can become utterly enchanted. If you watch a skilled dancer with culturally unacceptable proportions, you will experience a new freedom and beauty in your own body as you witness the truth: **every woman is beautiful.**

Beauty saves.

Beauty heals.

Beauty motivates.

Beauty unites.

*Beauty returns us to our origins,
and here lies the ultimate act of saving, of healing,
of overcoming dualism.*

~Matthew Fox

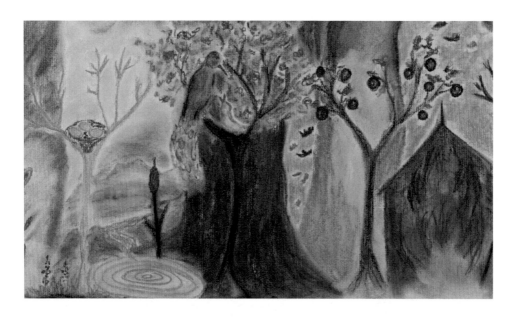

Bellydance for Your Body Parts

This is a simple sequence to get you started. As you deepen your dance practice, you will explore/ discover nuances in the dance of your body parts. Every part of you has intricacies and infinite details. Once you gain in skill, you can challenge yourself further by changing the sequence or combining isolations. For example, the hips do one thing, while the arms do another.

Put on some music that has some melody, but a strong beat:

Start with your head:
roll it, turn it, shake it, slide it, stretch your neck
Let this body part move through space,
responding in its own way to the music

Now move your shoulders:
roll them, pulse them, shake them, stretch them
Let this body part take you through space,
responding in its own way to the music

Then focus your attention on your spine:
wiggle, writhe, undulate, spiral
Follow the dance of the spine, and go where it bids you

Then dance with your hips: rock them, roll them, snap them, shake them, tilt and drop them.
Let this body part take you through space,
responding in its own way to the music
Discover new movements to delight you

And now focus on your *legs and feet*:
move the joints in dynamic ways, play with tempo and balance
Explore new ways of moving from this body part

Then put your attention into your *arms and hands*:
close your eyes and feel them move from the inside,
open your eyes and look at them as they trace mysterious designs
Follow the dance of wordless expression.

Now allow yourself some time
to flow through the body parts freely
Move from one body part to the next
in any order that expresses your music, your dance

5

Ancient Symbology

Before you can ever write a story, you must first learn to draw letters. In the first attempts at forming "O" or "B", is a sense of awe. Letters come from connecting curves and lines out of the utterance of sound.

This analogy works for learning dance, as well. In the art of bellydance, there is a set of foundational movements we will call the sacred shapes. Each shape is a symbol of an ancient wisdom; a connection to patterns inherent in all life.

Regard the shimmy for example. As the body vibrates, energy is stirred up and tension dissolves. Before people ever new about electrons or sound frequencies, they understood that the shimmy/shake hearkened to aliveness. Nowadays science confirms that all matter has an atomic vibration. A living body is a symphony of vibrational frequencies and patterns.

Once you can articulate these moving symbols, your body becomes a poetic expression of gesture. Our flesh and bones have a resonance with the sacred shapes. Not only do linear motions feel different from circular patterns, we actually create different biochemical reactions in our physiology with the movements we make.

"Cease trying to work everything out with your minds.

It will get you nowhere.

Live by intuition and *inspiration*

and let your whole *life*

be *REVELATION*."

– Eileen Caddy

Your Dance is a Sacred Gesture, a Moving Poem

Represented below is a pictorial image of the Ancient Symbols of Bellydance.

The foundational symbols of bellydance are the circle(O), the figure 8 (depicted horizontally), the undulation(S), and the shimmy (.(.(.).).). Four directions, spiral and hands are equally potent aspects of symbology, but not as common.

Refer to this drawing to connect with the shapes as they are described:

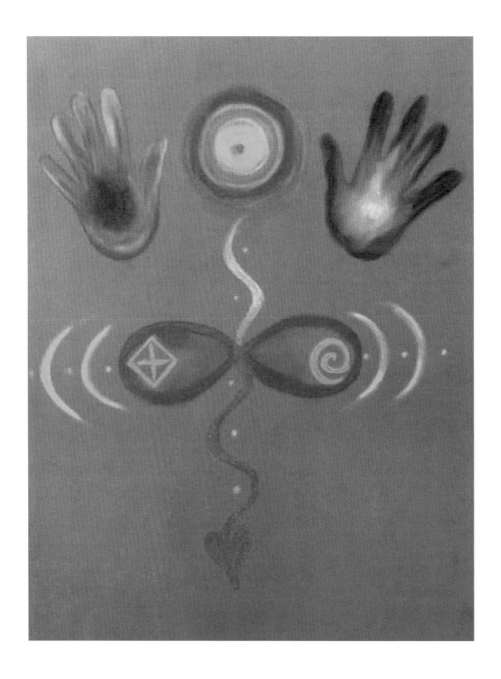

General Instructions for Dances of Sacred Shapes

The basic goal is to express all the sacred shapes in some way when you practice or perform. These shapes are playful and explorative. You let one shape travel around your body and into your space and then begin a new shape. It is very much like doodling with a pen and paper, but now in living, full-dimensional movement.

N.B. Take your time with these shapes. Each one is a full program in its own right. You could use a song for each one, or practise all of them within one song. Each sacred shape has manifold gems of wisdom. Explore them deeply and discover all the treasures latent in their dance!

Dance of the Circle

A drop creates a ripple

Circles radiate out

Ever expanding, spreading

Always connected, never ending

Circle of Life

Cycles

Wholeness, Oneness, Unity

Sun, Moon, Earth

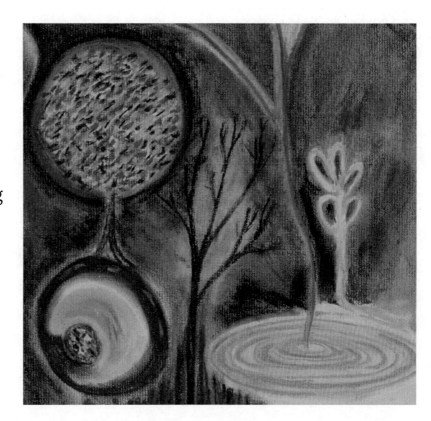

Draw various sizes of circles with your hips
Roll your shoulders, your head
Trace circular sculpture with your hands
Turn and spin in space
Change the tempo; moving fast and slow.
Sense how roundness and softness make you feel

Dance of Eternity (also known as 'Maia')

Figures of 8

Two opposites, joined at the centre

Duality

Symmetry

Carving, Massaging

Maia is the Mother of All

Womb of Chaos

Creative, Continuous and Complete

Sweep the air in large '8' patterns
Let the body sway in loops on the left and right, using the rib cage,
bringing them back to centre
The hips make the shapes in the horizontal and vertical planes
Can you find your full symmetry?
Can you invoke an off-balance '8'?

Dance of Undulations

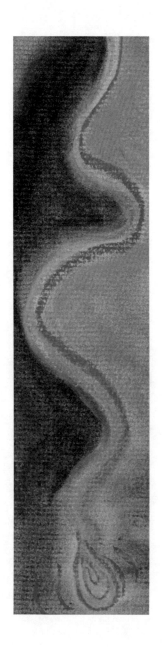

Snake

Wave

Light

Sound

Watery, Boneless, Sensual

Moving through matter

Carrying potency

Surrender your body to waving
Undulate the spine in snake-like movement
Writhe and pulse from the top of your head to your feet
Trace waves with the hands
Making swelling and subsiding waves with the arms,
like the movement on the ocean
Feel your breath as the waves expand and contract your chest
Feel the articulation of your joints as synovial fluids
bathe them in softness

Shimmy Dance

Ecstasy

Tremble

Vibration

Quickening

Catalyzing

Orgasmic

Shake it up

Shake it off

Shake it out

Begin to move your feet and hands as fast as possible
Let the energy gathering there travel up your limbs,
to your shoulders and hips
Allow the fleshiest parts of you to tremble and tickle
Let it travel deeper into your spine and then into your head
Your shimmy can become larger and 'out of control', crazy
and then soften and subside until it is a shimmer rippling your skin
Tap into the vibrational essence of all existence
Shimmy like the earthquake,
vibrato of the voice,
last sigh of life,
ecstasy of love

Tip: if you wear a coin belt on your hips, you will hear a shaking sound as you shimmy...

Spiral Dance

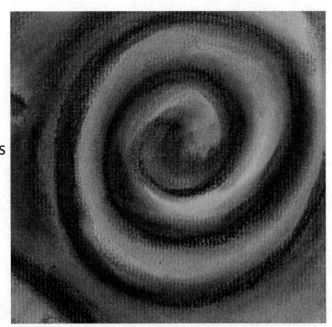

Patterns of Growth

From DNA and Bones, to Planetary Spheres

Expanding, Contracting

From the Infinite, Back to Home

A Mysterious Journey

Start from standing in stillness
Feel the space behind and below your bellybutton
Begin a circular motion,
allowing it to spiral and expand gradually, growing wider; bigger
When you reach the edge of the body with your feet rooted,
expand more
by lifting your feet and travelling in a spiral pattern through your space
When you reach the edge of the room,
begin to spiral gradually back into the centre
Be conscious of your pathway 'back home'
When you reach the centre of the room,
Continue spiralling inward by first spinning in the same direction
Then, contracting your energy and pulling the spiral inward,
until you are
returned to stillness

Dance of Direction and Lines

North, South, East, West

Vertical Up, Down

Horizontal Planes

Star

Square

Diamond

Triangle

Direct Lines

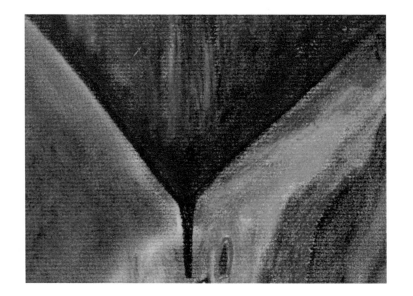

Move your arms in direct lines
Use sharp, staccato motions; no curves; up, down, here, there
Put a similar impulse in your legs; kick
Make out a point in the distance and travel directly to it
Create line geometry: stars, squares and triangles
Put this symbology into your chest; your hips
Feel the strength of directional dancing, the certainty, the contrast
Try to connect to the line that has no end, but extends to infinity
Send out an intention to that endless place, a wish, a prayer
Then close your dance in some way that feels appropriate to you

Hand Dance

The hands are special in Bellydance. They are more than a body part, and their 'shape' shifting is dance symbology at its essence; for the hands transcend definition. They can contribute to the dance in conscious ways, similar to ballet or other dance forms, but they have a deeper significance in bellydance; an ability to express mystery.

The hands are messengers of the soul. When a bellydancer allows the hands to articulate free patterns and gesture, they become a bridge of communication between worlds.

Sounds hokey pokey? If so, you may want to witness some other women (or children) dancing freely. Watch their hands. While the dancer is not fully aware of each hand gesture, they move or lie still in pure beauty. Notice what is revealed to you in their dance. The hands connect us to an otherwise invisible reality.

Try this:

As your chosen music plays,

Close your eyes and place your hands over your heart
Feel and sense your pulse and your breath
Allow the hands to move away from your heart and return at will
When you are comfortable with this,
allow your hands to dance around your body
Let them travel below your waist, above your head, in front,
behind and all around you
Where do they feel heavy?
Where do they feel the most free?
Do different sensations arise in different zones of your personal space?

Now, bring your hands, dancing before your face
Can you feel them stirring the air?
Move them to a comfortable position before you and open your eyes

Look only at your hands
Notice the shapes and movements of each finger,
the way your palm moves,
the softness of your wrist

Your hands are beautiful!
Magical!
Your hands are graceful, elegant, powerful and strong!

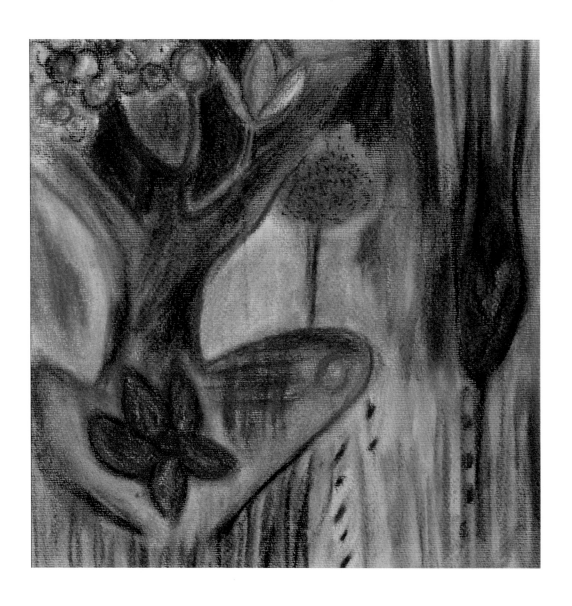

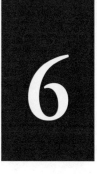

Menstruation:
Alchemy and Initiation

There is an enormous elemental force at work in women's bodies. It creates a repeated, yet fluctuating rhythm that is responsible for the creation of new life. Awareness of the flow of energy inherent in this cycle is vitalizing; creating a feeling of specialness and sweet intimacy.

With the onset of womanhood, a girl experiences menarche, her first bleed. It is a time to celebrate her initiation into the feminine mysteries; to share wisdom and knowledge, beauty and blessings. Laughter and love adorn her. Healing capacities and self-empowerment take root within her.

Like a wild genie (coming from the word 'Djiin' which means spirit), it emerges each month – disturbingly ecstatic, creative, restorative, and full of life. It 'speaks' of power, magic, and spiritedness. If we are willing to embrace the nature of our bodies, we are inducted into an intimate, yet universal source of 'knowing'. Rather than try to push the genie back into the bottle, we need to learn more about this spirit; to embrace it as 'genius'; something useful and powerful.

With the advent of menopause, the cycle shifts again, offering a woman access to deep pools of wisdom. Rather than being guided by her menstrual cycle, she becomes free to be the master of her genie and set her own ebb and flow through life.

Embodied within the culture of the bellydancer is a cyclical consciousness of the crimson thread that unites all women in feminine power. Bellydance cultivates a sense of nurturing and cradling of the uterus. Menstruation and menopause is welcomed and honoured with music, story, and dance.

For all women, the blood comes
as a reminder of the sacred feminine within.
Veiled within your womb
and within the ancient web
of mothers and sisters
is a wise and powerful goddess.
Listen to your belly.
Gather the women and celebrate.
-rephrased from a quote by Susun Weed

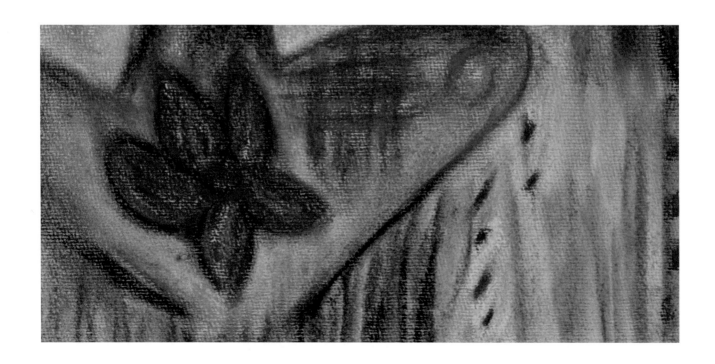

Embracing Change

The phases of menstruation correlate with other cycles of nature. There are four stages that repeat on a regular basis:

- Building the uterine 'nest' (follicular)

- Ovulation

- Determination (luteal)...(resulting in either releasing the egg or pregnancy).

- Bleeding

Each phase of menses can be likened to the 4 seasons and 4 elements.

Predicting your cyclical changes can help with planning and choices. For example, if you would like to do a fast, you may not want to begin it in the hungriest time of your cycle. If you are planning a home soiree, you may consider the sleepiest time of your cycle. Climbing a mountain is more challenging during the bleeding season of menstruation.

Charting your menses periodically is also a wonderful way to connect to your feminine cycle and discover bonds between body, mind and emotions. You may use the menstrual 'map' included in the appendix, or create your own.

N.B. If you are cycling through the menopausal years, you can cycle through the elemental seasons freely.

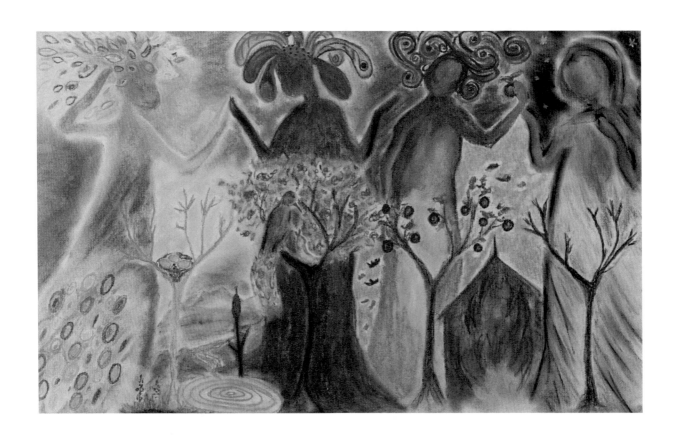

Tierra mi cuerpo (Earth my body)

Agua mi sangre (Water my blood)

Aire aliento (Air my breath)

Y Fuego mi espiritu (Fire my spirit)

~Ancient Women's Chant~

Dances of the Elements and Seasons

Welcome Air/Spring:

Air/Spring is the element of the East; connected to the soul and the breath of life. Air relates to sound, communication, wisdom or the powers of the mind. In spring, there are sonorous mating songs, the bubbling of newly-flowing waters and the chirping of babies. The air element carries away your troubles, blows away strife, and carries positive thoughts to those who are far away. Freshness and new possibilities come upon the breezes of air/spring. Air is associated with the colors yellow and white, and pastels, such as pink. Animals with feathers are air-element beasts. Fairy folklore invokes the air element. Music with wind instruments, such as flutes, will beckon your body into dancing light and airy.

For menstruation, air/spring is associated with the follicular phase. Here, the uterine 'nest' is prepared, and an egg is maturing. Like a seed, the chosen egg is nurtured and enhanced for release, while the uterus becomes engorged and nourished. This is the preparation for pregnancy. Our passions rise and we want to be 'busy as bees' and 'twitter-pated like the birds'. We become 'seekers': looking for what needs building, fixing, cleaning, creating.

Air/Spring Dance:

Playing music with flute

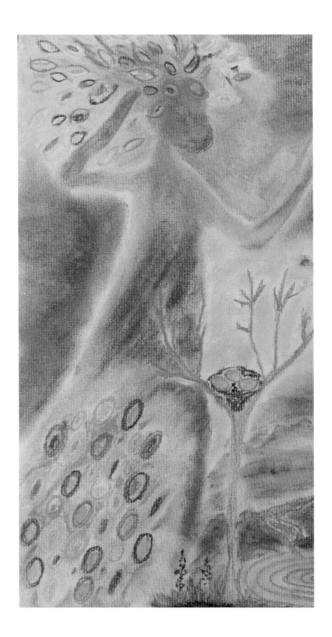

Breathe deeply and fully in your lungs,
making audible sounds

Imagine currents of air swirling around you,
and lifting you into space

Become like a leaf or a feather in the wind:
whirling and twirling about

The arms and hands are light and free, like
wings

Toss your cares to the breeze

If you like, you may pick up a veil and witness
the air dancing it

Welcome Earth/Summer:

Connected to the North, the Earth/Summer attribute is fertile and stable; nurturing; full of strength; solid and supportive. Yet, there is a hot and passionate core that bubbles under the surface. Thus, we see summer, bursting with color and sexual energy in all life. In the earth itself, this passionate nature results in volcanic explosions and lava flow. In color correspondences, use deep, rich greens, browns, and vibrant, flowery cousins of red, to connect to the Earth. In the body, our bones and organs of circulation are our earthly aspect. They provide structure and healing cells to support our life. Animals with fur are earth-element beasts. Gnome folklore is often about the spirit which cares for the earth. The music of the drum connects us to our earthly nature.

In the season of summer, there is a juxtaposition of celebration at the surrounding beauty, and an intense desire for rest. The temperature and plethora of colors and sounds invite us to lie upon the earth, and saturate our senses with splendor.

This can be compared to ovulation in the menstrual cycle. The uterus is ripe and full. As the egg is released and available for fertilization, there arises a heightened ability to 'conceive' within the mind and spirit as well as the body. A dual desire for initiating new ideas and dreaming without boundaries characterizes this phase. We become somewhat restless, but we also have a longing to be languorous and lazy. We want to linger in beautiful places such as gardens, adorned rooms, and dreams. When we surrender to the wellspring of the monthly visit of ovulation, and bask in the splendor of summer/earth energy, wisdom grows and bears fruit in our life.

N.B. It is wonderful to try a summery version of dance outdoors with the earth, when the dew covers the grass, or there is sand under foot.

Earth/Summer Dance:

Playing Music with Strong, Methodical Drum Rhythms:

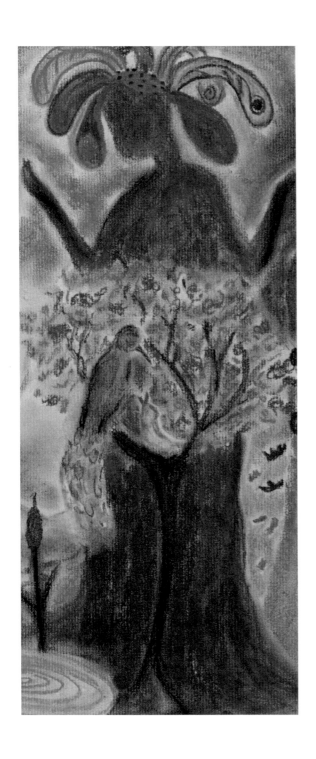

Begin in a crawling position,

the ground supporting your weight evenly

Connect to the earth through your hands and feet,

imagining the earth's molten core layers

Press and release the weight of your body through your limbs,

allowing the spine and hips to be subtle

Be aware of your bones

What animal natures come to mind for you in this moment?

Allow the movement of animals to strengthen you

and listen to that wisdom

Rise, keeping the beat of the drum in your feet and hips

Follow the impulses of your body

as you blend your movements to the music

Welcome Fire/Autumn:

Fire/Autumn has a purifying, volatile energy, associated with the South, and connected to strong will and energy. Fire/Autumn both creates and destroys. Fire can heal or harm, and can bring about new life or destroy the old and worn. Yellows and oranges and hot reds reveal that the Fire/Autumn season has come into the life cycle.

The Autumn season announces a transition into stillness, and a woman's response to this phase depends on her relationship to stillness. There can be fear and resistance. The dying leaves and colder times can feel like impending death. However, there can also be a wise welcome into the power of stillness and quiet. Inner warmth permeates this part of the cycle and a connection to a deeper fire (of spirit). In the body, the digestive system is connected to fire/autumn. Lizard-like animals with scales are associated with fire: snakes, lizards, salamanders.

In a woman's cycle, fire/autumn relates to the determination/luteal phase. The corpus luteum (shell of the egg) is either destroyed or maintained to initiate pregnancy. The egg's fate is determined by fertilization in this phase. This can be an emotional time in a woman's cycle, as hormones ebb and flow. Feelings and sensations intensify. There is urgency to complete projects and tasks. Often we become hungrier for food and other forms of nourishment. When at work, we can become overwhelmed with the immensity and sheer volume of the tasks. But if we choose our deeds and activities with honesty, we are rewarded with a harvest of wisdom and guidance.

Fire/Autumn Dance:

with some wildly chaotic music playing:

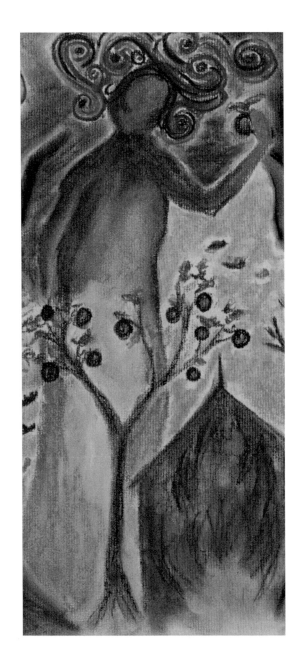

Initiate a shaking movement in your body
Shimmy and shake your hands, your legs, your hips
Move into chaos, dancing wildly, out of control
Burn up your stagnant emotions, move your
passions
Ignite your spirit
Dance as if you were flames, leaping, full of sparks

Welcome Water/Winter:

"I want to be like water.

I want to slip through fingers,

but hold up a ship."

~Michelle Williams

Used for healing, cleansing, and purification, Water/Winter is related to the West, and associated with moods and emotion; gentle rains, torrential downpours, misty mornings are all appropriate metaphors for feelings. In bellydance wisdom, water is the perfect balance of softness and power. We find this soft power when we regard the ocean or a cascade of water. Water flows over rocks, but can destroy them as well.

As you may expect, water/winter is associated with the color blue. Nymphs and undines are water elementals. Water dwellers all contain water wisdom. Watery music has a fluid melody; often slower in tempo. Frozen water comes to us as tiny, star-like crystals that we call snow.

The moon and its phases have influence upon the watery oceans and the menstrual cycle. Here we find the bleeding phase (or the early stages of pregnancy). This phase is introspective; a mirror and a gentle force of gravity. The quiet wisdom of water/winter requires us to settle into a serene, contemplative state of rest to be able to hear its subtle voice. A woman needs more sleep (or at least more time lying down and breathing deeply). She needs to reflect on what has come to pass. Prayer, meditation, dreaming, warm tea, meaningful conversation and long walks offer solace during this phase. Treating the blood of menstruation with a respectful or reverent gesture honours the life-giving energy that a woman carries forward each month.

Water/Winter Dance:

Playing music with a liquid feeling:

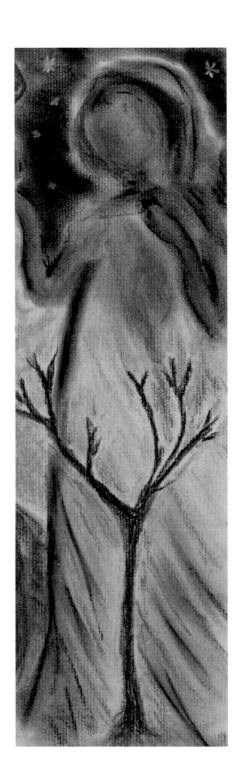

Soften your entire body,
Especially the shoulders, neck, spine and legs
Become so soft you have a sensation of water moving
over your skin and your bones undulating
Your arms and hands trace waves in space,
Tracing patterns of dancing waters:
Surging, swelling, rising and falling, rolling
Your spine writhes and ripples,
Cascading throughout your body,
Massaging your organs,
Bathing you with reverence

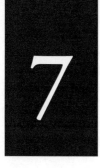

The Belly?

Bellydance is not all about the belly. However, the belly is central to creating the dance. The belly is always active. Movements are designed to affect the abdominal area; specifically, the muscles and organs which are cradled by the hips. The dancer's belly is framed by colourful cloth, jewels and sounds.

A bellydance practice enhances the power of the belly as a vessel of transformation. Fertility of all kinds is enhanced. Food is changed into life-giving energy. Babies grow there. Creative juices flow and ideas arise out of mysterious places; appearing as sensations of new life within the dance of the belly.

Your belly is a sacred chalice of life-supporting systems.

It's impulse is creativity.

The birth dance is particularly generative for creative inspiration. It celebrates the process of every potential conception as a birth; mimicking labor and delivery. Although it is therapeutic to do during pregnancy or to enhance fertility, the birth dance is also worth doing to ignite creativity and transformation in all aspects of your life.

"Whatever you can *do* or *dream* you can, **begin** it. Boldness has *genius*, power and *magic* in it!"

~ Johann Wolfgang von Goethe

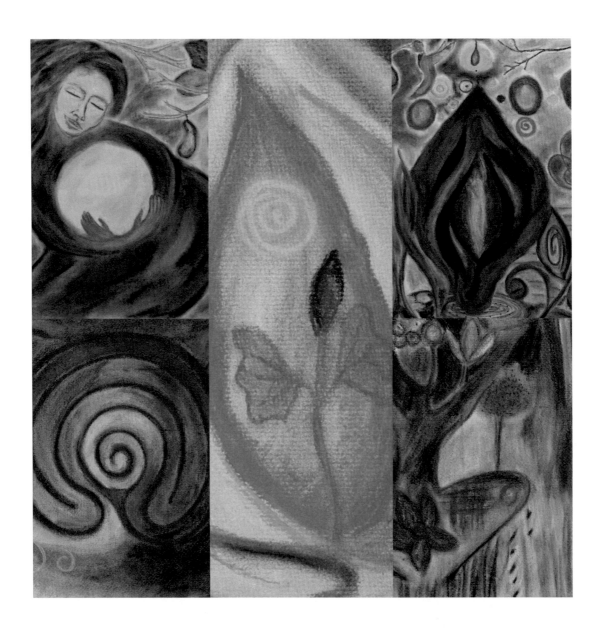

Try this:

Place your attention on your perineum
(These are the croissant-shaped muscles that form your pelvic floor)
Like the diaphragm located in the abdominal cavity,
your perineum is an organ of breath
The muscles are connected
to your reproductive passages and organs
Pull them inward and then allow them to soften and open fully
It is like moving an inverted lotus flower

Birthdance (with Veil)

Wrap a beautiful scarf over your entire belly
As the music plays, rub your belly as you soften your legs and feet
Breathe naturally as you allow your belly to relax and swell,
then diminish and contract inwards.
Use the muscles of your abdominals and spine
to create rolls and ripples in the belly.
After repeating this a few times, draw your attention
to the lotus of muscles in your pelvic floor
Like petals of a flower,
draw your pelvic floor upwards and relax it downwards
until you feel a warm softness there
Rub your belly again and massage that energy to your entire body with your hands.

Begin a squatting motion, opening the legs wide
Give the pelvis freedom to pulse and rock, sway and roll
Use strength to maintain this part of the dance as long as you can

Then allow your body to descend to the floor
Staying on your legs by kneeling in different ways, give freedom to your spine, head and arms
You can travel in space, but resist lying down for a time

Then descend further so that you are horizontal on the floor
Roll and writhe as if you were swimming
The arms, legs and head are free in space
The spine is supported by gravity and the transfer of weight in your body
In this dance, connect with your organs,
your internal dance of womb, intestine, liver, lung.
Massage these organs with your movements
Touch your entire body with your hands
Tickle, press, tap, squeeze

When you feel complete, allow stillness to come
Find a position of rest and comfort

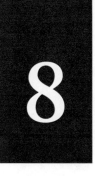

Happiness:
The Elixir of Life

Happiness is the magical elixir of a good life. A happy woman has a particular potency that cannot be found anywhere else. She radiates an energy that heals and influences whoever is in her presence. She cultivates a sacred grace that inspires greatness in others.

Men have said the following:

> *"A happy woman is like a slice of Heaven."*
> *"When I am with a feminine woman,*
> *it is like breathing fresh air."*
> *"My only aim in life is to make my wife happy."*

Ask the men in your life! You know that what I say is true. A happy woman radiates light in her eyes. Her skin is softer. She smells wonderful without perfume. Other people are happy just to be in her presence. A happy woman is a healing balm to suffering.

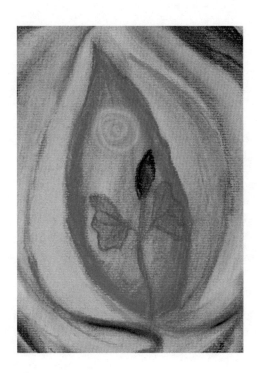

Become a Happy Woman.

...finding the tracks and traces

For the masculine, happiness is cultivated in production; having a purpose; a meaningful project; achieving results; meeting needs. For the feminine, happiness comes in unexpected delights; receiving little surprises; spontaneous infusions of gratitude. This feminine variety of happiness is a mystery. It is impossible to predict it; 'make' it happen; know its recipe.

A woman's happiness is like a slippery fish. It is so elusive that it is often hidden, even from herself as she seeks it. As a practice, try asking yourself the following question on a daily basis, "What is one thing that could be granted to me that would make me happy today?"

One thing is for sure, no one except you will 'know' how to make you happy. It is like tracking a well-hidden secret. There is no formula or guarantees. Happiness cannot be forced. What made you happy before may not make you happy today. That's why it is so magical and mysterious. That's why it is so special and worth pursuing.

"Don't ask what the world needs.

Ask what makes you come alive and go do it.

Because what the world needs

is people who have come alive."

~Howard Thurman

Rest and Play...essential ingredients

The first and foremost path to feminine happiness is abundant sleep. Just because we hear the cries of all the needs in our environment and have the ability for relentless multi-tasking does not mean we must/can do it all. Sleep is essential for a happy woman. Adequate rest puts you in a relaxed, receptive state where you can trace the fine pathway to what will guide you to happiness. So, if you are longing for a pillow and a blanket, GET IT and go to bed! Sleep makes you healthy, beautiful and energized, without drugs or lotion, and potions. It is a gift of 'happy', in and of itself.

The hormone that is abundant when a woman is infused with happiness is oxytocin. It commonly surges during sex and breast-feeding, infusing a sense of connection, trust and fulfillment in relationships. Slow, rhythmical movements such as swaying, massaging, washing, kneading and rocking also stimulate the production of oxytocin. In harmony with feminine physiology, the movements of bellydance originate in the work and play of women as they nurture and please their community of loved ones and themselves. Hence, bellydance is a sure way to self-fulfilling happiness!

So if you are rested and have some time to play, here is a little dance to get your happy juices flowing and put you on the path of glowing!

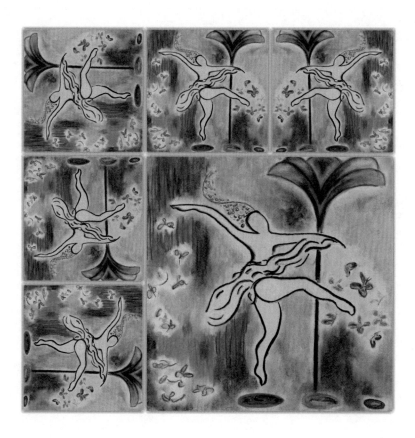

Happy Dance

Choose some music that invokes a perky, yet calm, mood:

Begin with your hands and move them through the air
Create painting movements, kneading motions, pulsations in your palms
Bring your hands to your body

Allow the hands to rub and massage you
as if you were spreading lotion over your skin
The hands travel to your belly, your thighs, your feet,
your breasts, your belly, your arms, your jaw and face
Spread loving care to all of yourself with a dancing caress
Adjust your position so that you can reach
and unwind all tension in the body
Now, beginning in your feet and softened knees, begin a little bounce
Allow the jiggles to come to your buttocks and thighs, belly and breasts
Allow the shoulders to relax and gently pulse with your bounce
Initiate a traveling movement: walking, skipping, and galloping
Try to travel with a bounce in your step
Pay attention to your breath and sigh deeply as you move
Bounce and jiggle, alternating your tempo

Follow Your Bliss!

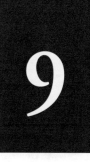

Daily Dance Bliss:
Getting In The Mood

Now that you have had a sample of dance experiences, you are ready to create your own pathways of dance in your life. A 'dancing lifestyle' is your life expression of spirit. As you penetrate wisdom, you can witness that verily, all life is a dance of emotion, relationships, and encounters of circumstance. Your breath; your bodily fluids; your passion; your instincts; your spirit; your feelings; are all dancing in your cells, organs and limbs! Images, thoughts and ideas are dancing in your mind! These life-dances can be conscious and peaceful or not, but they are your dances. Creating a dance practice will remind you that you are the Dance and the Dance of Life moves in you.

If you don't do your Dance,

who will?

~Gabrielle Roth

There will come times when you will not feel like dancing. Fatigue, illness, and inertia all interrupt our flow of motivation to do the things that restore and rejuvenate us. For this reason, it is useful to have a regular dance practice set into the rhythm of your life. Having a daily time and place for some dance creates a healthy habit that, even if it is interrupted, will easily return.

You're never too old to PLAY!

Dance 'Play' is a major component of the Dancing Lifestyle. Taking time to play with movement, music and other dancers is the way to keep our lives from being 'mundane' or 'routine'. When dance is a part of every day, life becomes a beautiful dance. Allow for small moments of dance to infuse your life.

" *Work* like you don't need the money.

DANCE like no one is watching.

Sing like no one is listening.

Love like you've never been hurt.

Live life every day as if it were your last."

~Irish Proverb

This chapter is an offering of dance catalysts. When you have had a break in your practice or your motivation wanes, try doing one of the little 'prescriptions for bliss' included in this chapter:

One Song, One Dance Every Day....

Take the time to dance with one song every day: just one little dance to a song that beckons you to move. That's all it takes to bring you into a state of connection, to lift your spirits, to get the blood and breath flowing. It's a moment of sanctuary, just for you....

Groovin' Inspiration...

It's easy to get your groove on!

First: Let your body choose a step that fits the music. Create some style with it.

Second: Choose two more steps to follow the first in succession. Move them your own, unique way.

Third: Return to the first move, and make it different somehow. Be expressive.

Allow the free-flow of steps and movement to come...there are no limits!

And remember: It's all about how it feels, not how it looks! Take a risk. Go to the edge of your comfort zone. Be willing to feel foolish. The glow of Beauty comes from Joy, Vulnerability, and Courage. When you find them in dance, you will find them in your mind and in your Life.

Mnemonic Inspiration...

Here is a little poetic phrase to help you play with movement in different ways. Begin with a sacred symbol (circle, 8, undulation, shimmy...see chapter 5 for more details). Go through the mnemonic, and create a new nuance to your movement to match that word. Remember: however you interpret the words will be 'right':

Reverse it, Revolve it
Profile it, Posterior it
Level it, Layer it
Tempo it, Texturize it
Size it, Send it
Travel it, Turn it
Fake it, Feel it

Props for Getting into Dance...

By taking an object into your dance-play, you will be able to let go of familiar patterns and create new relationships with your body and the ways it can move. If you don't have one of the props listed here, but wish you did...pretend. Your imagination can be the best 'prop' you have. Prop-ideas you can use in your dance sessions:

1.   Veils and scarves give a magical lightness to the dance. Cloth in the air can suggest birds, leaves, flames, swords, and magic wands.

2.   Balloons are also fun to dance with. Throw/catch, follow, wave them, and hold them with different parts of the body. Very fun!

3.   Objects you can balance on your body such as spoons, bowls, candle holders (with/ without fire), bean bags, sticks and swords challenge core strength, concentration, mobility and agility.

4.   Also try these props: hats, masks, dolls, ropes, chairs/stools, bells, tambourines and shakers. See what odd and innovative dances come to delight you.

10

Dance Gatherings:
Bellydance Bliss Together

We (women) thrive in community. It is relationship and connection that fosters our sense of safety. In a world that celebrates self-reliance and self-sufficiency, women have developed a multitude of talents and faculties. However, if we are so independent that we lose touch with our common ground, we become lonely and estranged. Activities such as bellydance (also singing, domestic activity and handwork), provide a social experience where women can connect to each other as distinctly female, regardless of their economic status, age, or family conditions.

Dance in a circle of women

Make a web of my life

Hold me as I spiral and spin

Make a web of my life

~song learned from Susun Weed

Traditionally, men were forbidden to participate or witness women's dance. This may seem exclusive, but there is wisdom in it. There is a sense of freedom when you can have fun without sexual tension. Women and girls of all shapes and sizes can enjoy each other's company and beauty while they wiggle and giggle! With only a few movements, they can have a good time; delighting in dance, needing no one.

In modern bellydance, a woman is free to dance how, where and when she wants, but she must also be conscious of the 'who, what, and why' it is all happening, if she is wise. The answers to these questions keep a dancer safe and powerful:

'Who is this dance for?'

'What is it saying/portraying?'

'Why am I dancing now?'

A women's circle creates an atmosphere of support and fun. The circle is a sharing place; a healing place; a sanctuary of nourishment, support and play. This chapter includes some fun games to enhance your dance gatherings.

The Ululation...freeing sound

An exciting sound to make at dance events is the ululation. It is a wild, high-pitched trilling sound that women make by moving the tongue rapidly up and down, or side to side. This sound has accompanied women in times of war and celebration. It is very powerful. To be modest, many women cover their mouth from view. To hear the sound, check it out on internet videos.

Collective Circle Dance:

Music is chosen with a familiar rhythm (crowd pleasing):

Forming a circle,
Each participant creates a short dance combination
She teaches it to the other participants in a chronological order
As music plays, each participant, in turn, does her combination
with the others following.

Veil Circle Dance:

Choose music that is flowing and lyrical. Select a veil that all participants can share:

One participant begins with the veil, dancing with it in the centre
All other participants move in harmony with the music,
maintaining and holding the perimeter
When done, the veil is offered to another participant
who enters the centre and dances
Continue passing until everyone has danced with it

N.B. Other props (or none at all!) could be used in a similar manner, such as candles, swords, feathers, clown noses, or anything you can think of.

Remember:

you are not performing for each other
you are sharing
you can talk while you dance
embrace moments of stillness
allow laughter and fun to infuse your efforts

Dance with a Music Challenge:

This one builds courage...give it a try, even if you don't think you can!

Each participant brings to the gathering a song that is special in some way.
It could be new, obscure, powerful, rhythmically challenging or simply a 'favorite'.

Participants take turns
offering themselves to dance to a completely 'unknown' song.
This is improvisation at its finest!
The dancer has the challenge of moving to music that she has not heard before, while connecting to the other participants.

There is no judgment whatsoever. It takes a lot courage to do this the first couple of times. After that, it might just become your favorite party game!

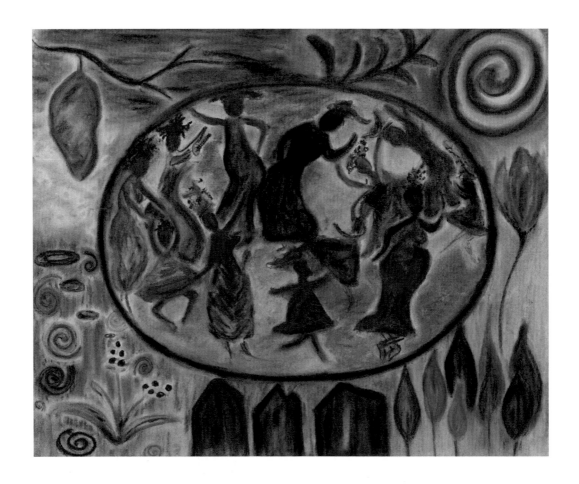

APPENDIX

Music is very personal, especially for a home practice. Truly, preferences are as diverse as our fingerprints. You can use any music that makes you wiggle and groove. However, many women love to have some suggestions to begin with. Here are some choices I have made to accommodate the dance inspirations. May you find your way through the myriad of musical landscapes that are currently available.

Chapter 1   'Full Circle' – Loreena McKennit

Chapter 2   (Touch) ' A Garland of Breath' – VAS

                    (Sight) 'At Siva's Feet' – VAS

                    (Hearing) 'Whispers of Rumi' – Dolphina

                    (Taste) 'El Desierto' – Lhasa de Sela

                    (Smell) 'Aphrodite's Mysteries' – Dolphina

Chapter 3   (Temptress) 'Leyli' – Cameron Cartio

                    (Mother) 'Hush-a-by' and 'Isabeau' – Connie Kaldor and Carmen Campagne

Chapter 4   'Astrae' – VAS or 'The Spirit We' – Rachel Sage

Chapter 5   'At Siva's Feet' – VAS

                    'De Cara a la Pared' – Lhasa de Sela

                    'She Moves in Mysterious Ways' – U2

                    'Kecharitomene' – Loreena McKennit

Chapter 6   (Air/Spring) 'Longing for the Unknown' – Karunesh

                    (Earth/Summer) 'Jilala: Nocturnal Ritual' – Moroccan Spirit

                    (Fire/Autumn) 'Huron Beltane Dance' – Loreena McKennit

                    (Water/Winter) 'Dance Dolphin Dance' – Dolphina

Chapter 7   'The Mystic's Dream' – Loreena McKennit

Chapter 8   'Blessings' – Solace

Chapter 9/10 'Ya Rayah' – Claude Challe
               'Eleni' – Johannes Linstead
               'Kalmady' – Mustafa Sandal
               'El Alem Allah' – Amir Diab
               'Wala Ala Baloh' – Nirvana
               'Marco Polo' – Loreena McKennit

Menstrual Map
– Alchemy of Wisdom-

This is a template for your use. You may wish to draw your own version. Add your personal touches: dates and length of each phase, your feelings, encounters, urges, images and associations. Notice the moments of expansion and contraction. As you chart your cycle throughout the year, notice patterns that arise and use your wisdom to harmonize your daily lifestyle/calendar in accordance with your cycle.

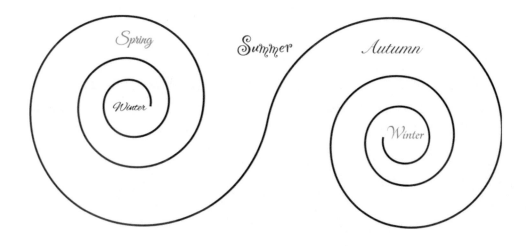

Sample of Menstrual Map

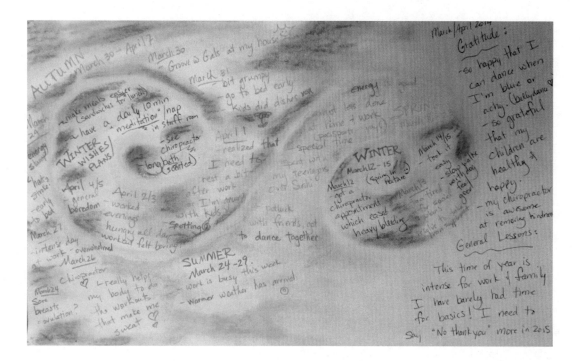

Acknowledgements

There is a blossom of gratitude for every insignificant breath and encounter that has brought me to this moment.

I would like to acknowledge Elaine and Monica of DanceEgypt for initiating me into this dance. The Baha'i's of Saskatoon and Regina deepened my understanding of unity in diversity and helped me feel my roots in the culture of humanity. The work of Alexandra Pope, Allison Armstrong and Flora Bowley have been huge influences in my life and this book. Every student who shared dance space with me deserves thanks for their queries and contributions to this study.

I would like to honour my father for planting the seed that I have something worth writing about. My husband and children deserve many hugs of gratitude for learning to live with a woman who is mildly outrageous and occasionally taken over by a creative muse.

I bow low for the contributions of my unofficial editors: Susan, Caroline, Anna, Beatrice and my mom.

May we all dance forever!

Printed in the United States
By Bookmasters